Pilates For Beginners

The Ultimate Guide to Mastering
Pilates for Beginners

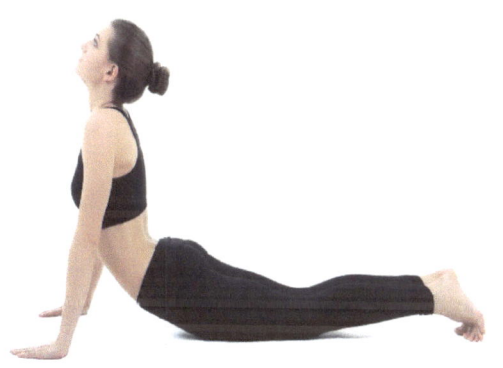

By
Fhilcar Faunillan

Fhilcar Faunillan

Table of Contents

INTRODUCTION

I want to thank you and congratulate you for downloading the book, *"Pilates for Beginners: The Ultimate Guide to Mastering Pilates for Beginners"*.

In this book you will learn what Pilates is all about and how it is a very good exercise for you. Also, you will learn about the basic information of Pilates, including its principle and simple exercise routines.

This book will also provide you steps and strategies in order for you to start your journey towards a healthier mind and body through Pilates. It is an easy and accessible way to train yourself into becoming the best you can be.

Thanks again for downloading this book, I hope you enjoy it!

Chapter 1 - History of Pilates

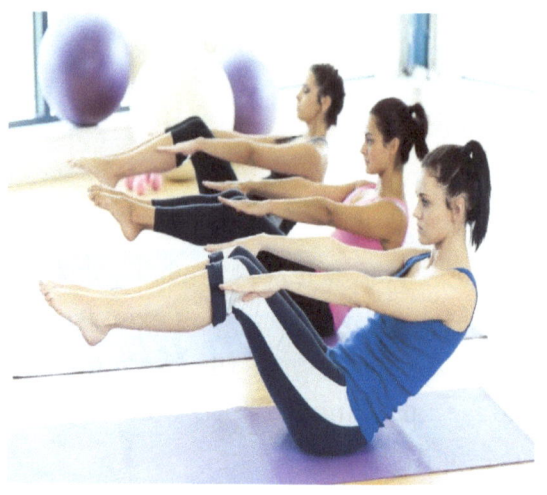

The amazing system of exercise, Pilates, was first designed by a physical-culturist from Germany named Joseph Pilates. His mother was a naturopath and his father was an award-winning Greek gymnast. During his lifetime, he studied both Western and Eastern forms of mind and body exercises to help him strengthen his body and overcome his ailments such as asthma. He was mainly influenced by the Greek ideal of a man who embodies a balanced mind, body, and spirit. For him to widen his knowledge, he did yoga, gymnastics, boxing, skiing, diving among other forms of exercises and even observed animals to learn how they move properly.

During the early part of the twentieth century, Joseph started to develop his own system of exercises. His main goal was to strengthen both the mind and body because he believed in the interrelation of physical and mental health. With the use of a variety of equipment he referred to as "Apparatus", he designed methods that helped people accelerate the process of strengthening, stretching, and aligning the body. He tried to devise several routines that will bring out the body's full potential.

In 1912, Joseph went to England and worked there as a self-defense instructor. During World War I, he was interned as an enemy alien together with other German Nationals. At the time of his internment, he trained the other internees with his system of exercise. At the time of the influenza epidemic in 1918 which killed thousands of people, none of Joseph's trainees died. After his release, he came back to Germany where his exercises gained favor especially within the dance community. Thanks to Rudolf von Laban who created a dance notation that is still popular until now. Joseph's exercises were also adopted by several dance curricula including the one by Hanya Holm. When the officials of the German government asked Joseph to train the army with his fitness system, he then decided to leave Germany for good.

In 1926, Joseph migrated to the United States where he met his partner Clara. Later on the two got married and together, they opened a fitness studio, which they named as "Studio for Body Contrology", in New York City. Among their clients were many New York dancers and ballerinas from the New York City Ballet. Dancers flocked into his studio after learning how Pilates is effective in creating a balanced, lean, and powerful physique. Joseph also had students who were famous boxers, opera singers, businessmen, war veterans, and many more. The Pilates exercise also became popular even outside New York as well. Hundreds of young students across the United States practiced this particular system of exercise too.

Joseph's students also began teaching his system of exercise making it more popular across the country. Two of them, Carola Trier and Bob Seed, opened their own studios and taught Pilates. Carola was a performing contortionist while Bob was a former Hockey player. Joseph and Clara were also friends to a lot of choreographers, including the famous George Balanchine.

When Joseph died in 1967, there was no line of succession for Pilates to continue. He had no will and designated no one to carry on his teachings. However, his partner Clara together with some of his students continued to operate his studio in New York. Around 1970, Romana Kryzanowska, who had studied with Joe and Clara, became the director. More and more of his students opened their own studios and taught Pilates as well.

In the 1980's the media started to cover Pilates. A lot of stars started to do the practice as well, making it more popular worldwide. Throughout the years, Pilates has entered the fitness mainstream. At present, millions of people all around the globe practice Pilates and the numbers are still increasing.

While there are already a number of excellent training programs that exist today, some of them produce inadequate instructors because of condensed and homogenous classes. Prices of trainings have also gone up ranging from $10-$20 per hour for mat-work exercises and $50-$100 per hour for utilization of Pilates equipment. Competent and well-trained teachers are important elements in achieving a student's full potential that is why in 2001, the Pilates Method Alliance was formed to support and maintain commitment to train instructors of Pilates. In 2005, the organization launched the Pilates Examination Exam to test a teacher's competency in teaching Pilates. At present, a lot of certified teachers are scattered all around the globe and more and more people are trying to embrace the standard of safety and competency in the practice.

Chapter 2 - What is Pilates?

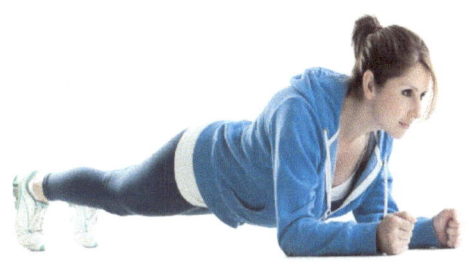

When you first hear about it, Pilates may seem to sound intimidating, but, you will eventually learn that it is an accessible method to achieve a healthier body. What exactly is Pilates? In Joseph Pilates' book entitlcd thc "Return to Life through Contrology", he described the Pilates method as an art of controlled body movements. When properly done or performed, this method should look and feel like a workout. It is composed of movements that enhance muscle strength, flexibility, and endurance. In this form of exercise, Joseph emphasizes the use of the lower back, hips, abdominals, and thighs. It also places emphasis on breathing, coordination, balance, alignment, and building a strong powerhouse.

Pilates is a focused and vigorous total-body exercise which makes use of a variety of spring loaded equipment. The Pilates system of exercise allows for modification and adjustments on the range of difficulty depending on the level of the student. It can go from beginner to advanced exercises depending also on the specific goals set by both instructor and student and also the limitations of those who practice it. As the person's body adapts to the activities, intensity can be increased through time.

With the use of systematic method of exercises paired with focused patterns of breathing, Pilates has proven itself over the past decades. It has become invaluable not in the field of fitness but has also become very useful in physical rehabilitation and professional sports training as well. As it was also widely embraced by the dancing community, the different exercises including "swan", "elephant", and the "pull navel to spine and then breathe" are now common amongst different classes, therapies, retreats, wellness centers, and even spas all across the globe.

From it being originally confined to a few people who practiced it mostly in a studio, Pilates has grown and was able to keep up with the needs of the modern times. With the increasing trend towards healthy lifestyles, Pilates is also used nowadays in schools and institution to teach the next generation fitness ideals. There are even a variety of modern schools of Pilates that are influenced by the physiotherapeutic approach to the method.

Contrary to the popular myth that Pilates was created for dancers and serious athletes, this exercise can be used and performed by everyone. While they are among the first groups that adopted this specific form of exercise, they are not the only ones who can benefit from it. As mentioned earlier, Joseph initially created this method for his own body improvement and also for his co-internees during the World War I. With this, it is important to note the Pilates is for everyone. This method will set your body for success, whether you goal is toning, training, or recovering, you will surely do better through time.

One must also know and understand that Pilates is different for everyone who practices it. When Joe taught this method back in the days, he was very specific according to the needs and capability of his clients. He would then modify the way the exercise was done depending on what each person's body needed. Therefore, there is really no right or wrong way to perform the Pilates exercises because it depends on the needs of the person doing it. Nothing is absolute so you do not have to worry if you do an exercise slightly different than how other performs it.

Another common misconception is that Pilates will always require the use of the specialized equipment called apparatus. Yes, when you think of the Pilates exercise you may probably visualize the reformer, an apparatus that looks like a bed frame with adjustable springs and a sliding carriage. But, the reality is that a lot of Pilates exercises can be done on the floor with the use of a mat. In fact, we can even refer to the mat-work as the purest form of Pilates. Joe created these exercises long before he began designing his apparatus. These mat exercises can be done anywhere and will probably take only

30 minutes per day. Back when Joe taught the Pilates exercise himself, every one of his client learned the mat and they were expected to practice it at home.

Pilates has something good to offer everyone, regardless of age and levels of fitness and ability. Joseph designed the apparatus to provide support especially for beginners and those people who have certain medical conditions. Also, the apparatus are built for people who want to further challenge their bodies and test its limits. Examples of this special equipment are the Reformer, the Wunda Chair, and the Cadillac. They are built with a system of strings and pulleys, handles and straps that can be adjusted according to the student's needs.

A typical routine of Pilates usually includes 25 to 50 repetitive strength training exercises. The Pilates method is somewhat considered similar to calisthenics which also uses push-ups and sit-ups as part of the training cycles. In fact, a lot of people refer to Pilates as the ultimate form of calisthenics. Pilates is a sensible and safe system of exercise that will definitely help you feel and look better. It teaches you a lot of things and has a lot of corresponding benefits not only to the body but to the mind as well.

Most of the workouts done in Pilates takes place with a person's spine laid flat, either facing up or down. The creator, Joseph Pilates, purposely used gravity in this manner to properly correct the different body imbalances which makes a person slouch and shrink from the proper posture. When the body is laid flat on the floor on top of equipment, the method then challenges the different muscles that serve as support to the spine through lifting the legs and arms, rolling up and down, arching, twisting, and bending, among others. It is important to remember that the key is to anchor the body to the floor and to stretch away from it. This creates opposition in the muscles which makes it strong.

Balance is also an important aspect in the practice of Pilates. The goal is to create a balanced and even body musculature in order to generate efficient patterns of movements. With this, the body can survive longer time of work without the risks of injuries because some areas maybe overused or underused. With proper balance, we can use all the parts correctly and accordingly so that we can reap all the vital benefits we can get from all the exercises.

Another thing you might notice in doing the Pilates workout is your core muscles which Joseph referred to as your "Powerhouse" or "Girdle of Strength". The muscles of your powerhouse include those that support your spine-- abdomen, inner things, lower back, and buttocks. We can say that almost all movements radiates from the center of the body. It is a goal of the Pilates exercise to strengthen these muscles in order to create a strong center in your body.

Pilates is a mind and body exercise that gives emphasis on the person's mental focus while performing different physical movements. It requires one to engage with the whole body while doing the different routines. At times, you strengthen one body part or muscle while stretching another. Pilates requires a lot of concentration because you cannot simply do the motions just like how you can move on gym equipment. This type of exercises gives weight to quality exercise rather than the quantity of movements performed. Instructors often try to coach on aspects such as the breathing quality, proper body alignment and posture.

Combining mind and body exercises helps better in the overall fitness of a person.

Let us try to consider one move in Pilates called the "rolling like a ball". This is done by balancing on your rear end, rolling backward, and then rolling back up into the initial position again. It may sound simple but it requires good balance and strength of the abdomen and lower back. Pilates helps you to be able to think on how you can use your muscles during exercise so that you can also use them better in your day to day routines. Through your developed focused in good posture, alignment, and body mechanics, you will then be able to sit and stand straight.

For a growing number of Pilates practitioners, it has become more than just an exercise method but a way of life as well. As the mind and the body is fused and reawakened, the Pilates method of exercise paves the way for a person to live a life where the gaps of thought and motioned are connected. No matter who you are or what condition you are in, Pilates helps enhance our daily life activities. Through it, we can then be able to manage our entire being and create positive connections with ourselves.

Chapter 3 - Principles of Pilates

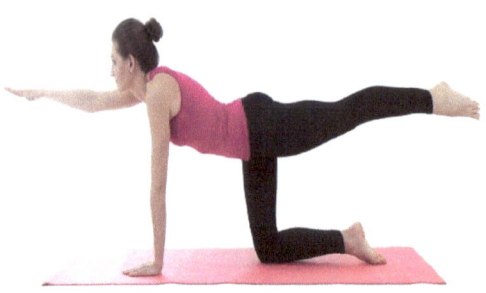

Joseph Pilates also called his method of exercise as contrology. In his book, he laid down several principles that help in defining his work better. These principles served as foundations for his approach to unify the body, mind and spirit. While the principles may seem abstract when taken individually, their integration will surely help a person in achieving grace, balance, and wellness.

Concentration

The principle of concentration concerns on how a person must bring full attention and commit to each exercise with the goal to get the most benefit from the workout. Pilates requires one to practice intense focus and concentrate on the task all the time. One must concentrate on the entire body during the duration of the workout for smooth movements. This may not be easy to do, but in the Pilates method, the ways the exercises are performed are more important than the exercises themselves.

Concentration is considered the mental key to attaining mind and body awareness. Proper concentration allows a person to do several repetitions of a movement without taking for granted other variables such as alignment and proper positioning.

Being mindful and focused can benefit us in a number of ways. Through concentrating fully on the task at hand, we are able to perform better. Concentration helps create a better connection between the mind and body and as one becomes more mindful of the body movements, one will be able to receive the maximum value that corresponds with it. Thus, optimum enhancement and body awareness is also achieved.

In creating an inner focus, your outward movements are affected as well. Say for example when you are in a crowded place on a busy day, you will be able to withstand all the people around you without being annoyed that much. Having a strong mind and body connection will allow you to react better to different situations in your day-to-day life.

Concentration also helps us notice where our body parts are and how each one of them is functioning. Also, it allows us to notice how these parts are in relation to each other and to the outside environment. This proprioception is very important both in the studio practice and also outside. To better understand this, think on how the exercises done in Pilates can be seen in the movements we do every day. Let us take for instance the movement called the sidekick series. We can see this movement evident when we walk or run. As we master this specific Pilates movement, we then become more aware of the functions of our hips making us walk and run more efficiently through time.

Precision

Precision is an essential element to correct Pilates. Each time you exercise, you must concentrate on doing the correct movements because when you do them incorrectly, you lose the vital benefits that come with the exercise.

In Pilates, there should be a focus in doing the perfect and precise movements rather than doing mediocre ones. Again, quality exercise is given more weight in this method of exercise. One should keep in mind that strength is best gained through few concentrated and correct efforts rather than a thousand sluggish ones.

As one goes deeper through the practice, each movement must then be executed with deliberate preciseness. Do not think much on how many repetitions you can make, instead, focus on trying to make each move as perfect as you can. Through proper awareness of the body, one is able to perform and sustain the movements properly. Remember that there are appropriate alignment and placement of each part relative to others.

By learning and appreciating how each body part play a very important role in our over-all functioning, we will become aware and also grateful on how our bodies work together to keep us moving every single day.

Control

The principle of control in Pilates is a result of a strong mind-body connection that is achieved through proper concentration and breathing. Joseph Pilates chose contrology as the preferred name for his method as it was based on the concept of muscle control. The main reason why you have to develop and practice concentration is to be able to take control of every aspect of each movement.

Control and precision are more concerned on how to do each movement properly to achieve effective and safe results rather than on the intensity or number of repetitions you can do. Proper control also allows you to stay within your body and keep up with the movements during the duration of the exercise. It is also important to remember that in Pilates, you should be in control of your body and not the other way around.

With proper control, you can utilize the correct form and do the exact movements leaving no part of your body unused. When you are mindful of all your actions, you direct each and every movement and take control over it.

This principle also extends so much more beyond the class or the studio. As we learn to control our bodies and become steady with our movements, we are able to avoid potential injuries. We are then able to carry ourselves in a safe and more graceful manner. Many injuries are caused by agitated and incorrect movements but with control and precision one can move more effectively.

Breathing

The principle of breathing is very essential in the Pilates method. In his book, Joseph devoted a large part of his introduction to breathing which he saw as the bodily house-cleaning with blood circulation. In here he explained how he saw the importance of increasing the intake of oxygen and its circulation to every part of the body. He considered this as a process of cleansing and invigoration.

Breathing is the process of deep and focused inhalation and exhalation that is done together with the different Pilates exercises. As mentioned, the Pilates method requires one to be aware with how the body works. Breathing is the important physical component that is necessary in attaining that level of awareness. With proper breathing, one is able to be at the moment.

Joseph teaches us to visualize the lungs as bellows when breathing and use them strongly to pump air in and out the body. You bring in air to the fullest when you inhale and release it in a similar manner. He even noted that breathing is the most integral part of every exercise and learning to breathe properly is the most important thing above all the others. He also emphasized the need to utilize a very full breath in doing the Pilates exercises.

The Pilates breathing is done through a posterior lateral breathing wherein one breathes deep into the back and sides of the rib cage. During exhalation, one must note the engagement of the muscles of the abdomen and pelvic floor. Pilates attempts to coordinate this breathing pattern with every movement of the method. In all the exercises, one is always instructed to breathe correctly above anything else.

Breathing is also a very useful principle in our daily lives because it reminds us to breathe properly and take deep and oxygenating breaths. As we all know, our breath basically sustains us in everything we do and every move we make.

The breathing principle also teaches us to be more aware of the things going on around whether it is emotional or physical. We become aware of it in deeper levels instead of just reacting directly to it. For instance, when you get into an argument with a person and he yells at you, the breathing principle helps you to take a deep breath and assess the situation properly before reacting to it. Thus, you get more time to think and respond appropriately to these kinds of situations.

Flow

The Pilates exercises are done in a steady and continuous flowing manner. Goals related to this principle are grace, ease, fluid and smooth movements which are all important in doing all exercises. The continuous and smooth movement during the transitions from one pose to the next will increase the strength and stamina of the person. During the exercise, the energy flows through the body evenly and connects all the body parts to attain proper integration. The Pilates apparatus, like the Reformer, is a useful equipment that mirrors flow and concentration.

Remember that the movements become easier if there are specific rhythms attached to it. The main goal of this principle is to maintain continuity in all the movements especially during several repetitions. Proper flow in Pilates helps one to improve performance and decrease chances of getting injured.

In our daily lives, the principle of flow teaches us to take like as it is. It allows us to accept life as it comes and moves through us each day. When we are "in the flow" or together with the flow, it means that move through life smoothly and with ease without being easily distracted by the different obstacles and diversions along the way. As we create flow and rhythm in our movements, we also create a smooth flow in our lives. Working with smooth transitions allows us to manage the different life transitions we face as well.

Our lives are filled with so many transitions and changes as we grow each and every day. Our daily activities require so much energy and if we do not learn to go through all these smoothly and negotiate it properly, wc may experience troubles along the way.

Centering
In the practice of Pilates, the starting point and source of the movements involved is the center of the body. As mentioned earlier, the Powerhouse is an important area which includes the muscles of the abdomen, lower back, pelvis, hips and glutes. Essentially, the exercises try to bring focus to the center of the body as it will calm the mind, body and spirit.

The energy being utilized is derived from the powerhouse, thus, it is only right to give emphasis and importance to this part of the body. It is the source of strength and stability for all the kinds of movement we make. For a practitioner to be able to control the body, he/she must always start at the center or the focal point.

Centering is helpful in our lives because it helps us understand the importance of our core and also teaches us to use it as a foundation for our movements. It aids us to become stronger and guides us to maintain form and alignment in the things we do. Being centered translates to being calm and balanced amidst the chaos and distractions that are present around.

If we are able to connect and utilize our powerhouse properly, we will feel more powerful and strong. At the same time, we will get the feeling of calmness that will help us avoid being out of control especially during situations that might put us to test. As we develop and maintain a strong center and correct posture, we can lessen the chances of injuring ourselves as we perform our daily activities.

Integration of the Principles

All these principles unite as one in order for the muscles to work properly and support all our movements. As you might notice, all the principles are interrelated with one another that is why it is important to remember that each one of them is important just like how each and every part of our body is important too. What we have to do is to learn on how to use all these parts and integrate them in unified movements in order to use our body's full potential.

Chapter 4 - Getting Started

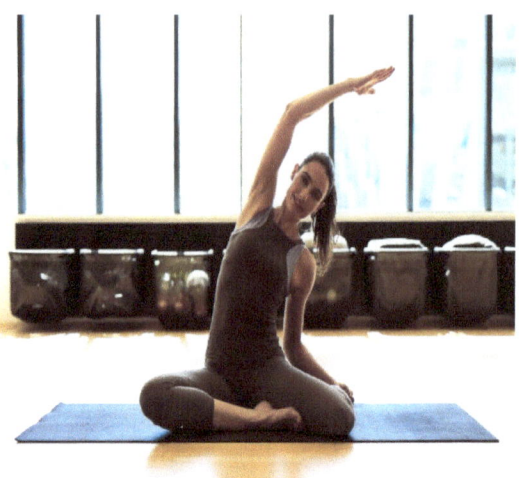

Once you have decided that you want to try Pilates, the next thing to ask would be, *"Where do I find Pilates?"*. To answer that, you may start looking for health and fitness clubs around you because a lot of them might teach classes such as Yoga and Pilates. Another option is that you might want to look for Pilates studios because these places are specifically geared towards teaching Pilates and it can guarantee you that they have the equipment needed for the optimum learning experience. You might also check at recreation, wellness and rehabilitation centers because they might offer sessions of Pilates as well.

As a beginner, it is important to choose the place which appeals best to you. You might want to adjust depending on your schedule, budget or comfort so choose a place that will best suit your needs. Just make sure that as a beginner, you might as well look for a place that can provide you the appropriate mind-body training and an atmosphere that is conducive for concentration and focus.

Before picking where to train, here are some things you might consider thinking about before getting into your final choice:

Pilates as a group experience vs One-on-one training

Based on your previous experiences or based on your personality, does working out with others help you perform better and keep you motivated? Do you need the presence of a lot of people to keep you enthusiastic about an activity and keep you on track? If yes, then mat classes or group reformer sessions may be the best choice for you. Many of the places mentioned earlier offer classes and even provide memberships for those who are interested. You can join together with your friends and colleagues so that you will find practicing Pilates more enjoyable.

If you want an intensive training, you can also inquire in the different studios or club if they offer one-on-one sessions. If you have the budget and if you really want to learn Pilates and exert full effort in it, then nothing beats personal training. With this kind of training, the instructor can be more focused in helping you do the movements properly. You can be taught and guided better because the attention is solely focused on you.

Finding the best class for you

In looking for a studio or place to practice Pilates, whether it is a group or personal session, consider the following things before getting started. First is that you make sure you choose a good mind-body environment that is dedicated to the practice of Pilates. Second, try to know if the place has good and experienced instructors. This is an important factor since they will be guiding you all throughout that is why you need people who know the field best. Next is that try to see if there are equipment available and if there is a wide variety of them. Also check the schedules of classes or sessions so that you can find what can suit you.

Practicing Pilates at home

If you prefer the privacy and solitude of working at home and you have a hard time sticking to class schedules, you can also choose to practice Pilates at home. If this method appeals best to you, you can hire a personal instructor or you can attend a few classes in your local studio or club then continue practicing at home. Experts say that attending a class or two is a safe and smart way to begin studying Pilates. You can learn the techniques and have the movements explained to you so that you can practice them properly on your own. You can design a small space at home so that you can use it for practice. If you have the extra money to get a qualified instructor, the better! In this way, you can get away with practicing with a group and you can stay more focused in the comforts of your own home.

Mat workouts

Pilates mat-work is popular for two main reasons: it is inexpensive and it requires lesser space. When you choose to stay at home, you can find a lot of instructional DVDs that can help you learn and improve. There are available variations ranging from beginner to advanced levels so you do not have to worry if you are just getting started. You can also buy additional accessories such as rollers and rings which can add challenge and variety to your workout.

Reformer workouts

Reformers are the most popular equipment used in the practice of Pilates. If you have the money, you can get yourself one so that your practice can be brought to a new level. With the system of ropes, springs and pulleys, the Reformer can provide both resistance and assistance in your workouts. This equipment allows you to expand the range of the variety of the different exercises and allows you to make them easier or more difficulty depending on your needs and goals.

Preparing for your first Pilates Class

The basic and fundamental Pilates movements and principles are all incorporated in the mat exercises. These are adaptable to any level, from beginner to advanced, so you do not have to worry about anything. It is important to learn the basics properly using the mat because it will help you gain strength and confidence in practicing Pilates. Later on, when you are familiar with the basics and ready to step up your practice, you will surely have fun using the different exercise equipment.

For your first class, you do not really need to bring than much with you. The studio usually provides for the things you need. But, some people might prefer to work-out using their own mats so you might also want to get one for yourself as well. Pilates mats are readily available in many local stores and you can also get one online. The studios might also sell them so you can ask around if they can offer you one.

Pilates mats are usually a little thicker as compared to the yoga mat. To be sure, you can ask your instructor first and seek out for recommendations. You might also want to bring a small towel with you and also a water bottle to keep you hydrated during the workout.

For the clothes to wear, there a few things you might want to consider in dressing for a Pilates class. First, you have to make sure that your clothes will allow you to move and stretch fully. Your alignment is also important and your instructor will check your posture from time to time so avoid using baggy clothes. Just the same as yoga, Pilates is done barefoot so there is no need for any shoes or fancy footwear. Also avoid excess accessories when you do workout, or they can be distracting and even dangerous especially when caught up in the different equipment you will be using.

Pilates terms you need to know

Abductor muscles - refers to the muscles that take the body parts away or farther from the midline of the body.

Adductor muscles - refers to as the muscles that take the body parts closer the midline of the body.

Core strength - the balanced and optimum development of both deep and superficial muscles of the trunk of the body .

Counter stretch - it is an exercise that allows the body to stretch in the opposite way the exercise before it was performed to somehow stretch the opposing muscles as well.

Diaphragmatic breathing - occurs when you take a deep breath into your belly using the muscles of your diaphragm.

Eccentric contraction - occurs when a muscle lengthens as it contracts to oppose a force.

Fitness Ball - also known as exercise, balance, and stability ball which aids in the different exercises making it more challenging especially in achieving a strong core.

Lateral Breathing - happens when one directs the breath into the sides and back of the ribcage.

Magic Circle - this is a flexible ring that is usually made of metal with paddled handles that are used to provide resistance during an exercise. It is popular in toning the chest, hips, arms and thighs.

Neutral Pelvis - this is an important reference point for Pilates exercises. When the pelvis is at its neutral point, the hip and pubic bones are in the same plane.

Neutral Spine - is a natural position when all the body parts are in good alignment.

Opposition stretch - this is a stretch where the body extends in opposing directions at the same time.

Pilates stance - this refers to a position wherein the legs are slightly turned out. The legs are rotated outward at the hip which leaves the toes apart and the heels together.

Pilates reformer - is an apparatus which consists of a platform that moves back and forth along a carriage.

"Scoop the abs" - is a phrase commonly used in Pilates which means to lengthen and deepen the abdominals toward the spine as if one tries to hollow out that area.

"Zip it up" - another commonly used phrase which means to drop the chest, pull in all the muscles of the abdomen, and then engage the pelvic floor.

Chapter 5 - Pilates Beginner Exercises

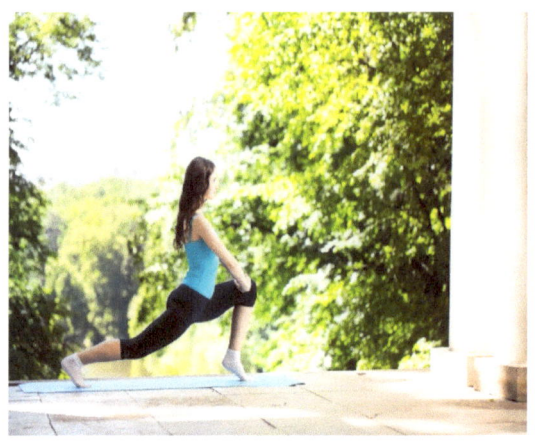

The following exercises are made easy to help you learn and familiarize with Pilates mat exercises. These exercises will help you achieve a strong core together with a stable and flexible body. You can do this on your own or if you choose to enroll under a class, have your instructor teach them to you according to your pace.

Warm-Up Exercises

In almost all other kinds of exercise, warm up is very important. In Pilates, it is an essential part in teaching the foundations of the method. It prepares the body for further movements making sure that it is safe to execute more challenging ones. A good warm-up before performing an exercise can help increase the body and blood temperature, dilate blood vessels, allow a more efficient cooling process, improve the range of motion and mentally prepare the person for the next activities.

A simple and typical warm-up may include jogging, stretching, simple calisthenics or flexibility exercises, among others. For a sample routine, you can do the twist warm-up exercise. First, find an area where you can do several strides. Start your warm up with simple skipping. Slowly add intensity, range of motion, and twists in each set. To further your warm-up, you may add arm swings, torso twists, and you may also drive your knees a bit higher. Make sure to keep your movements snap and controlled. It is up to you on how many strides you want to do as long as you add intensity to it gradually.

The Hundred

This is a classic Pilates mat-work exercise. Usually, you will be asked to do this at the beginning of any Pilates class you take. It requires you to coordinate movement and breathe as it warms up the lungs and the abdominal muscles. It may be challenging but modifications are available and if you are able to gain control, you will see the wide range of benefits it can offer.

To do the hundred, first lie on your back with your legs bent in tabletop position. Make sure that your ankles and shins are parallel to the floor. In here, you need to inhale. Next, exhale as you bring your head up while keeping your chin down.

Using the muscles of your abdomen, curl your upper spine up to the base of your shoulder blades. Scoop the abs, stay in this position, and then inhale again. At the same time, extend your arms and legs. Bring your legs according to what you can sustain and then exhale. Extend your arms just a few inches above the floor. Hold your position and take a few breaths. Repeat the cycle several times and do not forget to breathe.

Chest Lift

At first, this movement may seem like the abdominal crunch but it is important to note that the two are different ab exercises. The chest lift tries to create a deeper curve of the abdominal muscles down toward the mat which then results to a flat abs.

To do this, first lie on your back with the knees bent, legs parallel (with the knee, hip, and ankle in one line), and feet flat on the surface. Keep your shoulders down and then bring your hands behind your head and let the fingertips touch. Take a few breaths and check your body and make sure it is balanced side to side and relaxed. As you exhale, pull your belly towards the spine and allow it to lengthen. Tilt your chin slightly down and slowly lift the upper spine off the mat until the base of the scapula is just brushing of it. Inhale and draw the abdominals deeper. Exhale and keep the abdominals drawn in as you lower down the mat. Release the position and return to neutral spine. Repeat this and again, do not forget your breathing.

Roll-Up

This movement is also one of the classic Pilates mat-work exercises which is also known as one of the Pilates flat abs exercises. It greatly challenges the abdominal muscles and is said to be equal to six regular sit-ups.

To do the roll-up, first, lie flat on the floor with your legs straight. Allow your belly to drop down toward the floor and relax your shoulders making sure they are away from the ears. Breathe in and out and check your alignment. Also make sure that your scapula is anchored in your back and your ribs are down. Position your arms up over your head and back in a way where your fingertips are pointing to the wall behind you. Inhale, then leave your scapula down and bring your arms up over the head. Let your chin drop and the head, together with the upper spine, curl up to join the motion. Exhale and continue to curl your body "up and over" in a smooth motion toward your toes. Try to pull in your abs in and deepen the curve of the spine as you breathe in and out. Keep your head tucked, the back rounded, and the abdominal muscles deep as you reach for your toes. Inhale and then bring the breath fully into your back and pelvis as you try to pull the lower abs in. Then, reach your tail bone under and begin to uncurl, vertebrae by vertebrae, back to the floor.

Rolling Like a Ball

This classic Pilates mat-work exercise is also almost always included during a Pilates class. For some people, they can easily roll up like a pill bug and have a lot of find while doing so. On the other hand, for those who have low backs and find rounding difficult, this exercise might be a bit challenging at first. This move helps stimulate the spine, strengthen the abdominals, and tune the flow of our body's movement and breathing.

To do this exercise, first, you have to sit on your mat whole clasping your hands over your shins, just above the ankles. Then, drop your shoulders and widen your back. Also, make a nice curve in your spine and deepen your abdomen. Avoid tucking your head since your neck is part of that long curve. The next thing to do is to lift your feet of the mat and balance on your sit bones. Inhale as you pull in your lower abs in and up to get yourself going and then inhale as you try to roll back. Remember to roll only to the shoulders and not onto the neck. Exhale and stay scooped with your spine curved. Use your abdominals to return upright as you exhale. Balance yourself while doing this movement, repeat it for several times, and do not forget your breathing.

One-Leg Circle

This exercise is best in testing the strength of one's core. In order to do this, the abdominal muscle should work hard to keep the pelvis and shoulders stable all throughout the movement. It is a focus exercise and all the principles of Pilates are greatly seen in this movement.

To prepare, lie on your back with your back legs extended on the floor with your arms at your sides. Feel your body and balance the weight of your shoulders and hips on each side. To start, pull your abdominals in and anchor your shoulders and pelvis. Then, extend one leg towards the ceiling and lengthen it without lifting your hip. You may want to bend the knee slightly but make sure that your hips are stable and grounded on the mat. Inhale and then cross the extended leg to the opposite hip. Exhale as you drop it a few inches. Using control, open the leg out and sweep it around in a circular pattern back to the center. Do several circles in each direction and while doing so, breathe in and out.

Open Leg Balance

This movement is also one of the best in testing the strength of the lower abdominals and core. If you have a weak core, you will surely lose your balance in this pose. This pose also allows you to give your legs a good stretch and your back some extensions and stretching.

Perform the pose by starting in a sitting position. Then, try to bring your feet in toward your body keeping your knees open and feet together. Place your arms inside your legs and grasp your ankles making sure that the shoulders stay dropped. Next, pull in the abdominals and pay attention to lifting the lower abs as you extend one leg after the other. Try to balance and hold the pose for at least 5 counts. With control, slowly fold one leg after the other and bring them down one at a time.

Plank Pose

The plank is a well-known exercise that is also used in other fitness methods. It is a full body challenge that is popular in developing a stable frame and strong core. Plank may seem to be like a regular push up but instead of moving up and down, you remain positioned higher with your shoulders extended.

To do the plank, begin on your knees and place both hands in front of you with fingers grounded on the floor. Engage your abdominal muscles and lengthen your spine as you lean forward and align your shoulders with your wrists. Next, slowly extend your legs straight and keep them together. Hold the pose as you breathe deeply allowing he air to expand into your back and lower ribs.

The Side Kick Series

The exercises in this series are good for strengthening and toning the muscles of the hips, abs, and thighs. They try to give emphasis on length and use the powerhouse to stabilize the trunk as the lower body moves.

To set up, lie on your side with your shoulders, hips, knees, ankles, and ears aligned. Lift your ribs away from the mat so that the neck and back stay aligned. The front hand should rest on the mat in front of the chest. This can be used to help stabilize you but do not depend too much on it. Next, move your legs slightly forward to help you balance. Rotate the legs slightly in Pilates stance.

Kick Front
To do this, lift the top leg a few inches and then flex the foot. Then, swing the top leg to the front and at the full length of your kick try to do a pulse kick.

a)   Lengthen Back
While keeping the length of your leg, point your toe and move the leg to the back. Reach as far as you can but make sure not to move the pelvis and stay in this position for a while. After which, flex your foot and kick again towards the front.

b)   Side Leg Lifts
Inhale as you lengthen your body from tip to toe. Exhale as you use your core to bring both of your

legs up a few inches above your mat. Keep your inner thigs together. Inhale as your lengthen your legs back towards the mat.

c) Kicking Up and Down

From your set up position, also make sure that your abdominal muscles are pulled in and up. Then, lengthen the top leg as you kick up towards the ceiling. While doing this, make sure that the pelvis does not tilt back and the hipbones remains stacked. To move down, pull your abdominals up in opposition to the lengthening of your leg.

The Mermaid Side Stretch

This pose opens the sides of the body and lengthens the muscles governing its movements. It can be used as a gentle warm-up exercise or as a more intense movement in your routine as well.

To set up for the mermaid stretch, sit on the floor with both of your legs folded to the left side. Position the right hand flat on the floor to provide support and sit upright. Keep the other shoulder down away from your left ear as you try to extend the arm up above the head.

Lengthen and stretch to side while keeping your hip grounded. Extend your spine far up and take it to the other side. Remember not to let your ribs pop forward while doing so. To increase the stretch, move the support hand farther. You can even fold the support elbow to make it more intense. To return, use your abs to bring your torso up.

To stretch on the opposite side, bring the left arm down this time and use it as support. Extend the right arm and reach as far as you can without losing your shoulder's integrity. Return to the starting position after a few breaths by using your core.

Single Leg Stretch

This move trains the abdominals to move and initiate from the center. It also helps develop a strong support and stabilize the trunk as the limbs are in motion.

To prepare, lie on your back with your knees bent and shins parallel to the floor. Breathe in and out in this position. Then, pull your abs and curl your shoulder and head up to the tips of the shoulder blades. While doing this, extend the left leg at a 45 degree angle. Keep the other leg in the initial position and grasp the right ankle with the right hand. Also move the left hand to the right knee and maintain the upper body curve all throughout. Switch legs this time, now with the left hand holding the left ankle and the right hand on the left knee. Switch the legs for several times and release if you are already feeling so much tension in your neck and shoulders.

Spine Stretch
The spine stretch is a great exercise for the hamstrings and the back muscles. It is useful in almost all kinds of workouts as it prepares you for more challenging exercises.

To start, sit tall with your legs extended shoulder width apart. Inhale and extend both your arms in front, shoulder height. Exhale and try to lengthen your spine and curve forward reaching your toes. Inhale and reach a little further as much as you can. Exhale and return to the initial position by using your lower abdominals.

Double Leg Stretch

The double leg stretch is a very good ab workout that draws strength from the powerhouse and demands great endurance from the core.

To do this exercise, first curl up. Lie on your back with shins parallel to the floor. Pull in your abs and curve your upper body as you grasp your ankles or shin. Reach long and extend your limbs in opposite directions. Keep your abs pulled in and your lower back grounded on the mat. Then, pull back into center and curl up again. Do not drop the curve and keep your chest and head lifted. Do the extension and pulling back to center several times and remember to keep yourself aligned to center.

The Saw

The saw is designed for back and hamstring stretch. It is a good way to experience opposition stretch and as you grow to be familiar with it, it becomes very interesting as you work with the oppositional dynamic between your different body parts.

To start, sit up straight on your sit bones and extend both legs in front. Stretch your arms to the side even with your shoulders. Inhale as you turn your whole torso keeping your hips even still. Exhale as you follow your back hand as you turn your upper torso as if you are curling yourself. Stretch as you try to reach the fingers of one hand across the opposite foot. Once you are able to extend as much as you can, hold the position and then inhale returning to sitting. Repeat the exercise on each side and do not forget to keep breathing while doing so.

The Swan

The swan is considered an extension exercise as it tries to help you counter stretch after a lot of forward flexions. It opens the anterior part of the body and gives the chest and abdomen a good expansion and stretch. In addition, it also strengthens the shoulders, back, thighs, pelvis, glutes, hamstrings and abdomen.

To do this pose, lie on your mat faced down and keep your arms close to your body. Then, try to ben your elbows to bring your hands under your shoulders and make sure they are away from the ears. Also remember to keep the legs together. Next, engage the muscles of your abdomen. Inhale as you lengthen your spine and press your forearms and hands into the mat to create a long upward arc in the upper part of the body. Exhale as you keep lifting the abdominals. Release the arc, lengthen your spine and slowly return onto the mat. Repeat this pattern for several times.

Pilates Push-up

The Pilates push-up is an advanced way to do the push-ups. It is very good in developing the core and arms. Also, it is best for strength, stability, and endurance training.

To begin, do the standing position with the correct Pilates posture. Bring your arms up straight over the head. Bend your body as you try to get your hands onto the mat. Walk out to a plank position and make sure to keep your shoulders away from your ears. Then, pause at the front plank position for a while as this helps stabilize your shoulders. Next, lower down toward the mat, just like doing a regular push-up. Return to plank, walk back, and roll up again to standing position.

Chapter 6 - Benefits of Pilates

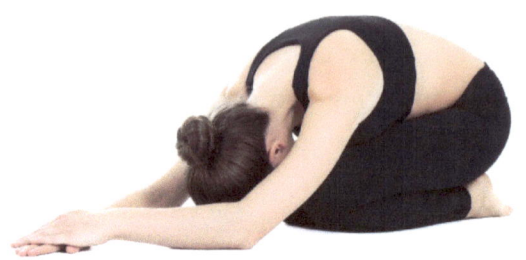

Practicing Pilates comes in with a lot of great benefits not just for the body, but for the mind as well. By creating a strong center and through the application of the principles in Pilates, you will surely see loads of good effects including the following:

Body awareness

Perhaps, one of the greatest benefits of doing Pilates is that you become aware not just of your body but also to the present. When Pilates has become part of your lifestyle already, you will see how things become easy especially when you do them in the right manner. Pilates changes your shape as it teaches you the ways of daily living. It allows you to train not just your body but your mind as well through concentration and control.

Better flexibility

The different Pilates exercises lengthen and tones the muscles of the body. As you reach further into each pose, you squeeze the juice out each time you exercise. When you engage all your parts, you are helping them to become more flexible. At first, you may feel some strain after doing some exercises but as you practice more and more, you will see how you can get passed through what you thought as your body's limits.

A strong core

One of the main goal of Pilates is to develop a strong core or center as it is one of the foundations of all the other movements of the body. As you go through the exercises, you then develop strong core which can lead you to have a good shape as well.

Increased height

Our everyday activities contribute to the compression of our spine that leads to loss in height. As we grow old, our spine also compress that is why without exercise we may be at risk for some bone malfunctions. To counter these effects, Pilates gives importance to posture, alignment, and centering. With the help of exercise, your muscles are strengthened and you are lifted up in a better posture.

Grace and control

The principles governing Pilates make sure that the benefits you can get will be very useful in your daily live. As you improve your movement, coordination and awareness, you will learn more about your body and how it moves. Also, you will gain control not just over your actions but your thoughts as well.

Better brain function

As mentioned, Pilates requires you to focus and pay attention to what you are doing. You are using your mind all throughout the routine and you are exercising it as well. A lot of research suggest that when you use your mind and think on what you are doing, there is an increase in the growth rate of brain cells. Your nervous system creates better connections all throughout your body making it function better.

Helps prevent injuries

As you learn to do things correctly and with grace, you will see that the risk for injuries decreases. Your body stays balanced and conditioned that is why you do not have to worry about getting sprains. You are able to move better with ease in all the things you have to do every day.

Weight Loss

Pilates is an activity that works out the muscles of your body. It can also be very helpful in developing a good structure and maintaining a healthy weight as well. Paired with proper diet, you can definitely achieve a good weight in doing Pilates. Classes can vary according to intensity so if you want to shred of a lot, you can ask the instructor to adjust your workouts.

Confidence

Beyond all the physical benefits of doing exercise, one of the rather rewarding things you get is confidence in yourself. When you are able to use your body to its full potential you will start to feel good about yourself. When you are able to do the things you thought were once impossible, you will get the sense of fulfillment. You will feel more healthy and vibrant on the outside as the inner energy radiates all throughout.

Chapter 7 - Additional Tips and Reminders

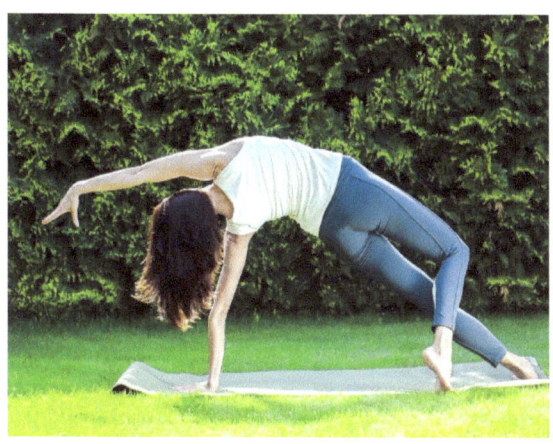

For beginners, it is important to know the basic things about Pilates in order to learn it in the correct manner and avoid injuries along the way. Here are some additional tips and reminders you can use in the practice of Pilates.

1.   Attend trial classes

Before you sign up for a studio or club, you might want to attend a few trial classes or walk in classes to see if you will feel comfortable with the environment and the instructors. In this way, you can go from place to place and see what suits you best.

63

2. Warm-Up is Necessary

In almost all activities, may it be sports or exercise, warm up is essential to center and prepare oneself for strenuous activities. Pilates is not only a physical activity but it trains the mind as well that is why you need to be prepared every time you start a class. Take a few minutes to listen to your body and prepare it together with your mind as well.

3. Safety first

Safety is very important in Pilates, and in a lot of other workouts too. It is important to follow instructions properly. If there are modifications and protocols needed to be done in order to assure your well-being, follow it. Before starting a class you might want to check yourself for injuries. If you have several problems, consult it first to avoid further complications. Talk to your instructor if you have any concerns so that he can adjust according to your needs. Do not try to impress others by doing so much more than your body allows you to because you might end up having a broken neck for that.

4.   Always protect your Neck and Upper Spine

In doing the exercises, make sure that you do it properly according to the instructions and have your teacher assist you if you do not understand a few things. Make sure your neck and upper spine are protected. If you need to, you can make use of a neck roll or a pillow to support these parts.

5.   Low legs make more challenge

If you want to challenge yourself in a pose, you can lower your legs because this will make your abdomen work harder. As you practice, you can adjust it depending on how much you want to test yourself.

6.   For those who have tight hamstrings

Do not worry if as a beginner you have tight hamstrings and find it difficult to do several exercises. You can always use a folded towel or foam to lift your hips slightly higher to support you. You can also bend your knees slightly if you find the poses hard already

7.   Never forget to breathe

Breathing is again very essential in the practice. As you do the different movements and poses, never ever forget to breathe. Do not hold your breath for too long because this will prevent the proper flow of nutrients in your body. At first, you might find it hard to keep up but with practice, concentration and perseverance, you will notice that everything will be smooth as you go on every time.

8.   Do not forget to have fun while doing exercise

The element of fun should never be taken for granted. You become better at what you do especially if you enjoy doing it that is why remember to have fun when you are exercising. At first, it may be tiring but just think of the corresponding benefits you will get if you pursue and push yourself towards your limits.

CONCLUSION

Thank you again for downloading this book!

I hope this book was able to help you learn and understand the basics of the Pilates method. Pilates is a very good mind and body workout that will surely help develop your full potentials. The next step upon successful completion of this book is to get your own mat and find the nearest Pilates class to you. Do not wait for long because you need to work your body out so that you will become healthy and fit.

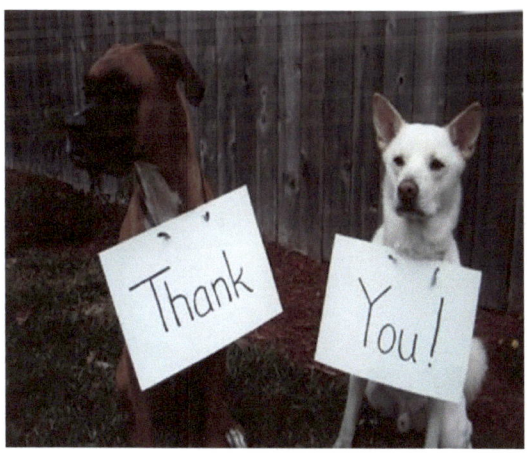

Finally, if you enjoyed this book, then I'd like to ask you for a favor, would you be kind enough to leave a review for this book on Amazon? It'd be greatly appreciated!

Thank you and good luck!